VEGAN COOKBOOK FOR TYPE 1 DIABETICS

Delicious Plant-Based Meals for Managing Type 1 Diabetes

T. John

COPYRIGHT PAGE

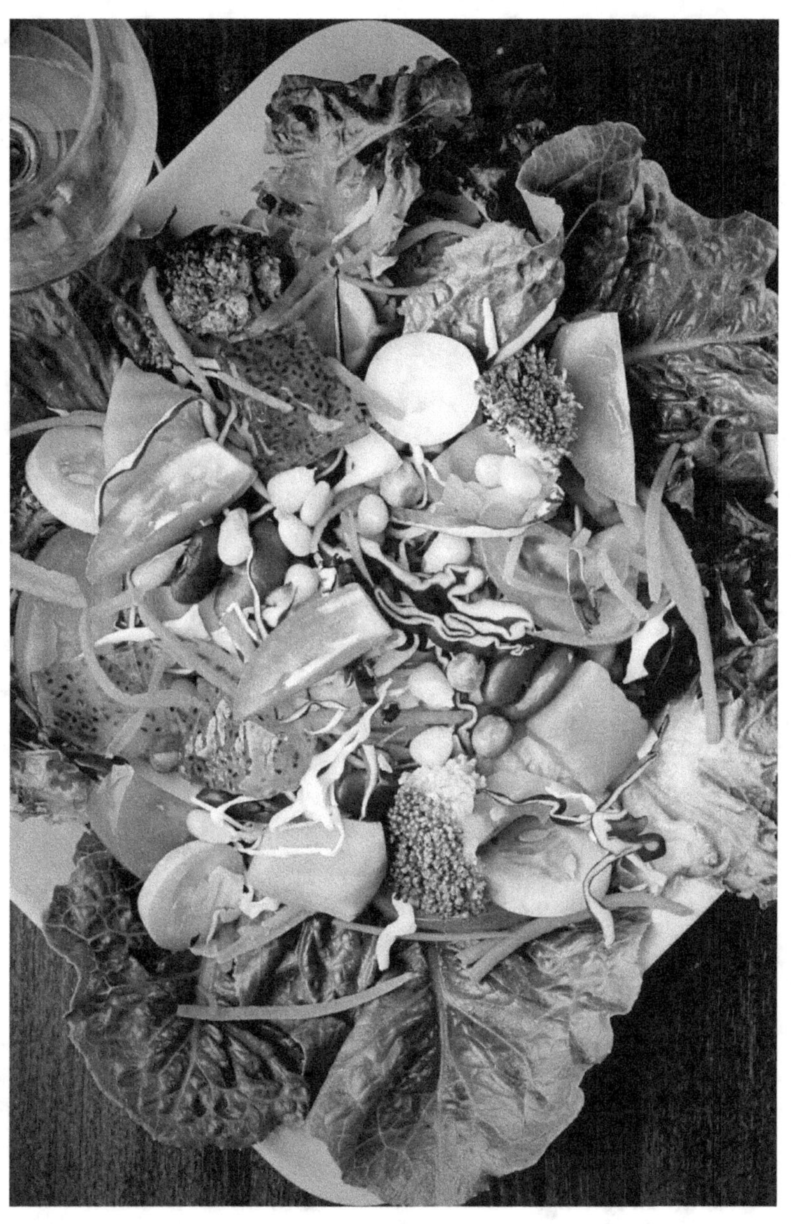

TABLE OF CONTENTS

Chapter 3: Lunch Recipes.....................44

Chapter 4: Dinner Recipes 69

Chapter 5: Snacks and Appetizers 94

Chapter 6: Desserts 114

Chapter 7: Smoothies 138

CONCLUSION 154

INTRODUCTION

I magine your body as a complex ecosystem, where sugar (glucose) acts as the fuel for your cells. Type 1 diabetes disrupts this delicate balance. The pancreas, responsible for producing insulin, the key that unlocks the cellular door for glucose entry, malfunctions. This leaves excess sugar circulating in the bloodstream, leading to a myriad of health issues.

How Plant-Based Power Can Benefit Type 1 Diabetics

While there's no magic bullet, a well-planned vegan diet can be a game-changer for type 1 diabetics. Here's why:

- **Fiber Fiesta**: Plant-based meals are bursting with fiber, the slow-digesting superhero. This translates to steadier blood sugar levels, preventing those dreaded spikes and crashes.
- **Weight Management Marvel**: Vegan diets tend to be lower in calories and saturated fat, promoting

healthy weight management. Maintaining a healthy weight can significantly improve insulin sensitivity.

- **Cardiovascular Champion**: Vegan diets are naturally cholesterol-friendly, reducing the risk of heart disease, a common complication of diabetes.

Blood Sugar Management

Living with type 1 diabetes requires a proactive approach. Here are some tips to keep your blood sugar in check:

- **Carb Counting Comrade**: Become familiar with carbohydrate counting, a technique that helps predict blood sugar response to food. This allows you to fine-tune your insulin dosage for optimal control.
- **Teamwork Makes the Dream Work**: Collaboration is key. Work closely with your doctor and a registered dietitian to create a personalized meal plan and insulin regimen.
- **Exercise Enhancer**: Regular physical activity is your diabetes BFF. Exercise improves insulin sensitivity and overall well-being. Find activities you

enjoy, whether it's a brisk walk, a dance session, or a yoga flow.

- **Blood Sugar Monitoring Buddy**: Regularly monitoring your blood sugar levels empowers you to make informed decisions about diet, exercise, and insulin adjustments.

Embrace the Journey:

Living with type 1 diabetes can feel daunting, but you're not alone. By exploring the potential of a vegan diet, mastering blood sugar management techniques, and working with your healthcare team, you can thrive on this journey.

Chapter 1: 30 Day Meal Plan

Week 1:

Day 1:

- Breakfast: Quinoa Porridge with Berries
- Lunch: Lentil Soup with Spinach and Carrots
- Dinner: Lentil Bolognese with Zucchini Noodles
- Snack: Guacamole with Baked Tortilla Chips
- Dessert: Vegan Chocolate Avocado Mousse

Day 2:

- Breakfast: Tofu Scramble with Spinach and Mushrooms
- Lunch: Chickpea Salad Sandwich with Whole Grain Bread
- Dinner: Chickpea Curry with Brown Rice
- Snack: Hummus with Carrot Sticks and Celery
- Dessert: Banana Ice Cream with Almond Butter Drizzle

Day 3:

- Breakfast: Chia Seed Pudding with Almond Milk
- Lunch: Quinoa Salad with Roasted Vegetables
- Dinner: Vegan Chili with Quinoa and Kidney Beans
- Snack: Edamame with Sea Salt
- Dessert: Berry Crisp with Oat Topping

Day 4:

- Breakfast: Vegan Pancakes with Sugar-Free Fruit Compote
- Lunch: Vegan Caesar Salad with Tofu Croutons
- Dinner: Eggplant Parmesan with Marinara Sauce
- Snack: Roasted Chickpeas with Spices
- Dessert: Vegan Cheesecake with Strawberry Sauce

Day 5:

- Breakfast: Avocado Toast with Tomato and Basil
- Lunch: Stuffed Bell Peppers with Brown Rice and Black Beans
- Dinner: Teriyaki Tofu Stir-Fry with Vegetables
- Snack: Sliced Cucumber with Lemon and Tajin
- Dessert: Apple Cinnamon Energy Bites

Day 6:

- Breakfast: Breakfast Burrito with Black Beans and Salsa
- Lunch: Greek Salad with Tofu Feta Cheese
- Dinner: Spaghetti Squash Pad Thai with Tofu
- Snack: Vegan Cheese and Crackers
- Dessert: Pumpkin Spice Oat Bars

Day 7:

- Breakfast: Overnight Oats with Apples and Cinnamon
- Lunch: Mushroom and Spinach Quesadilla with Whole Wheat Tortillas
- Dinner: Stuffed Portobello Mushrooms with Couscous and Spinach
- Snack: Trail Mix with Nuts and Dried Fruit
- Dessert: Chocolate Chip Chickpea Cookies

Week 2:

Day 8:

- Breakfast: Green Smoothie Bowl with Kale and Pineapple

- Lunch: Vegan BLT Wrap with Tempeh Bacon
- Dinner: Vegan Shepherd's Pie with Mashed Cauliflower
- Snack: Avocado Salsa with Whole Grain Crackers
- Dessert: Coconut Mango Sorbet

Day 9:

- Breakfast: Sweet Potato Hash with Peppers and Onions
- Lunch: Thai Peanut Noodles with Tofu and Broccoli
- Dinner: Mexican Quinoa Stuffed Peppers
- Snack: Stuffed Mini Bell Peppers with Vegan Cream Cheese
- Dessert: Lemon Poppy Seed Muffins

Day 10:

- Breakfast: Vegan Breakfast Casserole with Tofu and Vegetables
- Lunch: Cauliflower Crust Pizza with Vegan Cheese
- Dinner: Ratatouille with Polenta
- Snack: Caprese Skewers with Cherry Tomatoes and Basil

- Dessert: Peanut Butter Banana Cookies

Day 11:

- Breakfast: Banana Walnut Muffins
- Lunch: Black Bean and Corn Salad with Lime Dressing
- Dinner: Jackfruit Tacos with Mango Salsa
- Snack: Baked Sweet Potato Fries with Chipotle Aioli
- Dessert: Raspberry Chia Seed Jam Bars

Day 12:

- Breakfast: Coconut Yogurt Parfait with Granola
- Lunch: Baked Falafel with Hummus and Pita Bread
- Dinner: Butternut Squash Risotto with Sage
- Snack: Spinach Artichoke Dip with Whole Wheat Pita Chips
- Dessert: Almond Butter Cups with Dark Chocolate

Day 13:

- Breakfast: Spinach and Tomato Breakfast Quesadilla
- Lunch: Sweet Potato and Black Bean Burrito Bowl

- Dinner: Cauliflower Alfredo Pasta with Peas and Mushrooms
- Snack: Vegan Spring Rolls with Peanut Dipping Sauce
- Dessert: Blueberry Coconut Popsicles

Day 14:

- Breakfast: Vegan French Toast with Maple Syrup
- Lunch: Spinach and Mushroom Quiche with Tofu
- Dinner: Veggie Stir-Fry with Quinoa
- Snack: Roasted Vegetable Platter with Balsamic Glaze
- Dessert: Carrot Cake Energy Balls

Week 3:

Day 15:

- Breakfast: Blueberry Almond Smoothie
- Lunch: Vegan Sushi Rolls with Avocado and Cucumber
- Dinner: Vegan Gumbo with Okra and Brown Rice
- Snack: Seaweed Snacks with Wasabi Peas
- Dessert: Vegan Rice Pudding with Cinnamon

Day 16:

- Breakfast: Quinoa Porridge with Berries
- Lunch: Lentil Soup with Spinach and Carrots
- Dinner: Lentil Bolognese with Zucchini Noodles
- Snack: Guacamole with Baked Tortilla Chips
- Dessert: Vegan Chocolate Avocado Mousse

Day 17:

- Breakfast: Tofu Scramble with Spinach and Mushrooms
- Lunch: Chickpea Salad Sandwich with Whole Grain Bread
- Dinner: Chickpea Curry with Brown Rice
- Snack: Hummus with Carrot Sticks and Celery
- Dessert: Banana Ice Cream with Almond Butter Drizzle

Day 18:

- Breakfast: Chia Seed Pudding with Almond Milk
- Lunch: Quinoa Salad with Roasted Vegetables
- Dinner: Vegan Chili with Quinoa and Kidney Beans
- Snack: Edamame with Sea Salt

- Dessert: Berry Crisp with Oat Topping

Day 19:

- Breakfast: Vegan Pancakes with Sugar-Free Fruit Compote
- Lunch: Vegan Caesar Salad with Tofu Croutons
- Dinner: Eggplant Parmesan with Marinara Sauce
- Snack: Roasted Chickpeas with Spices
- Dessert: Vegan Cheesecake with Strawberry Sauce

Day 20:

- Breakfast: Avocado Toast with Tomato and Basil
- Lunch: Stuffed Bell Peppers with Brown Rice and Black Beans
- Dinner: Teriyaki Tofu Stir-Fry with Vegetables
- Snack: Sliced Cucumber with Lemon and Tajin
- Dessert: Apple Cinnamon Energy Bites

Day 21:

- Breakfast: Breakfast Burrito with Black Beans and Salsa
- Lunch: Greek Salad with Tofu Feta Cheese

- Dinner: Spaghetti Squash Pad Thai with Tofu
- Snack: Vegan Cheese and Crackers
- Dessert: Pumpkin Spice Oat Bars

Week 4:

Day 22:

- Breakfast: Overnight Oats with Apples and Cinnamon
- Lunch: Mushroom and Spinach Quesadilla with Whole Wheat Tortillas
- Dinner: Stuffed Portobello Mushrooms with Couscous and Spinach
- Snack: Trail Mix with Nuts and Dried Fruit
- Dessert: Chocolate Chip Chickpea Cookies

Day 23:

- Breakfast: Green Smoothie Bowl with Kale and Pineapple
- Lunch: Vegan BLT Wrap with Tempeh Bacon
- Dinner: Vegan Shepherd's Pie with Mashed Cauliflower
- Snack: Avocado Salsa with Whole Grain Crackers

- Dessert: Coconut Mango Sorbet

Day 24:

- Breakfast: Sweet Potato Hash with Peppers and Onions
- Lunch: Thai Peanut Noodles with Tofu and Broccoli
- Dinner: Mexican Quinoa Stuffed Peppers
- Snack: Stuffed Mini Bell Peppers with Vegan Cream Cheese
- Dessert: Lemon Poppy Seed Muffins

Day 25:

- Breakfast: Vegan Breakfast Casserole with Tofu and Vegetables
- Lunch: Cauliflower Crust Pizza with Vegan Cheese
- Dinner: Ratatouille with Polenta
- Snack: Caprese Skewers with Cherry Tomatoes and Basil
- Dessert: Peanut Butter Banana Cookies

Day 26:

- Breakfast: Banana Walnut Muffins

- Lunch: Black Bean and Corn Salad with Lime Dressing
- Dinner: Jackfruit Tacos with Mango Salsa
- Snack: Baked Sweet Potato Fries with Chipotle Aioli
- Dessert: Raspberry Chia Seed Jam Bars

Day 27:

- Breakfast: Coconut Yogurt Parfait with Granola
- Lunch: Baked Falafel with Hummus and Pita Bread
- Dinner: Butternut Squash Risotto with Sage
- Snack: Spinach Artichoke Dip with Whole Wheat Pita Chips
- Dessert: Almond Butter Cups with Dark Chocolate

Day 28:

- Breakfast: Spinach and Tomato Breakfast Quesadilla
- Lunch: Sweet Potato and Black Bean Burrito Bowl
- Dinner: Cauliflower Alfredo Pasta with Peas and Mushrooms
- Snack: Vegan Spring Rolls with Peanut Dipping Sauce
- Dessert: Blueberry Coconut Popsicles

Day 29:

- Breakfast: Vegan French Toast with Maple Syrup
- Lunch: Spinach and Mushroom Quiche with Tofu
- Dinner: Veggie Stir-Fry with Quinoa
- Snack: Roasted Vegetable Platter with Balsamic Glaze
- Dessert: Carrot Cake Energy Balls

Day 30:

- Breakfast: Blueberry Almond Smoothie
- Lunch: Vegan Sushi Rolls with Avocado and Cucumber
- Dinner: Vegan Gumbo with Okra and Brown Rice
- Snack: Seaweed Snacks with Wasabi Peas
- Dessert: Vegan Rice Pudding with Cinnamon

Chapter 2: Breakfast Recipes

In this chapter, we've curated a collection of delicious vegan breakfast recipes that are not only diabetes-friendly but also packed with flavor and wholesome ingredients. From hearty porridges to energizing smoothie bowls, there's something here to suit every palate and dietary need.

Quinoa Porridge with Berries

Ingredients:

- 1/2 cup quinoa
- 1 cup almond milk
- 1/2 teaspoon cinnamon
- 1/4 cup mixed berries
- 1 tablespoon chopped nuts (optional)

Instructions:

1. Rinse quinoa under cold water.
2. In a saucepan, combine quinoa, almond milk, and cinnamon.

3. Bring to a boil, then reduce heat and simmer for 15-20 minutes until quinoa is cooked and mixture is creamy.

4. Serve topped with mixed berries and chopped nuts, if desired.

Nutrition Information:

- Calories: 250
- Protein: 7g
- Carbohydrates: 40g
- Fat: 6g
- Fiber: 6g
- Sugar: 4g
- Portion Size: 1 cup

Tofu Scramble with Spinach and Mushrooms

Ingredients:

- 1/2 block firm tofu, crumbled
- 1 cup spinach, chopped
- 1/2 cup mushrooms, sliced

- 1/4 teaspoon turmeric

- Salt and pepper to taste

Instructions:

1. Heat a non-stick skillet over medium heat.

2. Add crumbled tofu and cook for 3-4 minutes.

3. Stir in spinach, mushrooms, turmeric, salt, and pepper.

4. Cook for another 3-4 minutes until vegetables are tender.

5. Serve hot.

Nutrition Information:

- Calories: 180

- Protein: 15g

- Carbohydrates: 8g

- Fat: 10g

- Fiber: 3g

- Sugar: 2g

- Portion Size: 1 serving

Chia Seed Pudding with Almond Milk

Ingredients:

- 1/4 cup chia seeds
- 1 cup almond milk
- 1 tablespoon maple syrup
- 1/2 teaspoon vanilla extract

Instructions:

1. In a bowl, whisk together chia seeds, almond milk, maple syrup, and vanilla extract.
2. Let sit for 15 minutes, then whisk again to break up any clumps.
3. Cover and refrigerate overnight.
4. Serve chilled with your favorite toppings, such as fresh fruit or nuts.

Nutrition Information:

- Calories: 180
- Protein: 4g
- Carbohydrates: 15g
- Fat: 10g
- Fiber: 10g

- Sugar: 4g
- Portion Size: 1/2 cup

Vegan Pancakes with Sugar-Free Fruit Compote

Ingredients:

- 1 cup whole wheat flour
- 1 tablespoon baking powder
- 1 tablespoon flaxseed meal
- 1 cup almond milk
- 1 tablespoon apple cider vinegar
- 1 tablespoon maple syrup
- 1 teaspoon vanilla extract
- 1 cup mixed berries

Instructions:

1. In a bowl, whisk together flour, baking powder, and flaxseed meal.
2. In a separate bowl, mix almond milk, apple cider vinegar, maple syrup, and vanilla extract.

3. Combine wet and dry ingredients, stirring until just combined.

4. Heat a non-stick skillet over medium heat and pour batter to make pancakes.

5. Cook for 2-3 minutes on each side until golden brown.

6. Meanwhile, heat mixed berries in a saucepan until soft and juicy.

7. Serve pancakes with warm fruit compote.

Nutrition Information:
- Calories: 220
- Protein: 6g
- Carbohydrates: 40g
- Fat: 4g
- Fiber: 6g
- Sugar: 8g
- Portion Size: 2 pancakes

Avocado Toast with Tomato and Basil

Ingredients:

- 2 slices whole grain bread
- 1 ripe avocado
- 1 medium tomato, sliced
- Fresh basil leaves
- Salt and pepper to taste

Instructions:

1. Toast whole grain bread until golden brown.
2. Mash avocado and spread evenly on toast.
3. Top with sliced tomato and fresh basil leaves.
4. Season with salt and pepper to taste.

Nutrition Information:

- Calories: 280
- Protein: 7g
- Carbohydrates: 22g
- Fat: 18g
- Fiber: 10g
- Sugar: 2g
- Portion Size: 1 serving

Breakfast Burrito with Black Beans and Salsa

Ingredients:

- 1 whole wheat tortilla
- 1/2 cup black beans, drained and rinsed
- 2 tablespoons salsa
- 1/4 avocado, sliced
- Fresh cilantro, chopped

Instructions:

1. Warm tortilla in a skillet or microwave.
2. Spread black beans and salsa on tortilla.
3. Top with sliced avocado and chopped cilantro.
4. Roll up tightly and serve immediately.

Nutrition Information:

- Calories: 320
- Protein: 10g
- Carbohydrates: 40g
- Fat: 12g
- Fiber: 12g
- Sugar: 2g
- Portion Size: 1 burrito

Overnight Oats with Apples and Cinnamon

Ingredients:

- 1/2 cup rolled oats
- 1/2 cup almond milk
- 1/4 cup unsweetened applesauce
- 1/2 teaspoon cinnamon
- 1 tablespoon chopped walnuts

Instructions:

1. In a jar or bowl, combine rolled oats, almond milk, applesauce, and cinnamon.
2. Stir well to mix all ingredients thoroughly.
3. Cover and refrigerate overnight.
4. In the morning, stir oats and top with chopped walnuts before serving.

Nutrition Information:

- Calories: 250
- Protein: 7g
- Carbohydrates: 35g
- Fat: 10g

- Fiber: 7g
- Sugar: 8g
- Portion Size: 1 serving

Green Smoothie Bowl with Kale and Pineapple

Ingredients:

- 1 cup kale leaves, stemmed and chopped
- 1/2 cup frozen pineapple chunks
- 1/2 ripe banana
- 1/2 cup almond milk
- 1 tablespoon chia seeds

Instructions:

1. In a blender, combine kale, frozen pineapple, banana, and almond milk.
2. Blend until smooth and creamy.
3. Pour into a bowl and sprinkle chia seeds on top.
4. Enjoy immediately with a spoon.

Nutrition Information:

- Calories: 200
- Protein: 5g
- Carbohydrates: 35g
- Fat: 6g
- Fiber: 8g
- Sugar: 15g
- Portion Size: 1 serving

Sweet Potato Hash with Peppers and Onions

Ingredients:

- 1 medium sweet potato, diced
- 1/2 bell pepper, diced
- 1/2 onion, diced
- 1 tablespoon olive oil
- Salt and pepper to taste

Instructions:

1. Heat olive oil in a skillet over medium heat.

2. Add sweet potato, bell pepper, and onion to the skillet.

3. Cook, stirring occasionally, until sweet potato is tender and lightly browned.

4. Season with salt and pepper to taste.

5. Serve hot.

Nutrition Information:

- Calories: 220
- Protein: 3g
- Carbohydrates: 30g
- Fat: 10g
- Fiber: 6g
- Sugar: 8g
- Portion Size: 1 serving

Vegan Breakfast Casserole with Tofu and Vegetables

Ingredients:

- 1 block firm tofu, crumbled

- 1 cup diced vegetables (bell peppers, mushrooms, spinach, etc.)
- 1/2 cup nutritional yeast
- 1/2 teaspoon garlic powder
- 1/2 teaspoon onion powder
- Salt and pepper to taste

Instructions:

1. Preheat oven to 375°F (190°C) and lightly grease a baking dish.
2. In a bowl, mix together crumbled tofu, diced vegetables, nutritional yeast, garlic powder, onion powder, salt, and pepper.
3. Transfer mixture to the prepared baking dish and spread evenly.
4. Bake for 25-30 minutes until set and lightly browned on top.
5. Serve hot, garnished with fresh herbs if desired.

Nutrition Information:

- Calories: 180
- Protein: 15g

- Carbohydrates: 10g
- Fat: 8g
- Fiber: 4g
- Sugar: 2g
- Portion Size: 1 serving

Banana Walnut Muffins

Ingredients:

- 1 1/2 cups whole wheat flour
- 1 teaspoon baking powdcr
- 1/2 teaspoon baking soda
- 1/4 teaspoon salt
- 3 ripe bananas, mashed
- 1/4 cup maple syrup
- 1/4 cup almond milk
- 1/4 cup chopped walnuts

Instructions:

1. Preheat oven to 350°F (175°C) and line a muffin tin with paper liners.
2. In a bowl, whisk together whole wheat flour, baking powder, baking soda, and salt.

3. In another bowl, mix mashed bananas, maple syrup, and almond milk.

4. Combine wet and dry ingredients, then fold in chopped walnuts.

5. Spoon batter into muffin cups and bake for 20-25 minutes until golden and a toothpick inserted into the center comes out clean.

6. Let cool before serving.

Nutrition Information:

- Calories: 160
- Protein: 4g
- Carbohydrates: 25g
- Fat: 6g
- Fiber: 4g
- Sugar: 10g
- Portion Size: 1 muffin

Coconut Yogurt Parfait with Granola

Ingredients:

- 1 cup coconut yogurt
- 1/2 cup homemade or store-bought granola

- 1/4 cup mixed berries

Instructions:

1. In a glass or bowl, layer coconut yogurt, granola, and mixed berries.
2. Repeat layers until ingredients are used up.
3. Serve immediately as a nutritious and delicious breakfast option.

Nutrition Information:

- Calories: 300
- Protein: 6g
- Carbohydrates: 40g
- Fat: 14g
- Fiber: 6g
- Sugar: 12g
- Portion Size: 1 serving

Spinach and Tomato Breakfast Quesadilla

Ingredients:

- 2 whole wheat tortillas
- 1 cup spinach leaves
- 1/2 cup cherry tomatoes, sliced
- 1/4 cup vegan cheese, shredded
- Salsa for serving (optional)

Instructions:

1. Heat a non-stick skillet over medium heat.
2. Place one tortilla in the skillet and layer spinach, tomatoes, and vegan cheese on top.
3. Place the second tortilla on top and press down gently.
4. Cook for 2-3 minutes on each side until golden brown and cheese is melted.
5. Cut quesadilla into wedges and serve hot with salsa if desired.

Nutrition Information:

- Calories: 280

- Protein: 10g
- Carbohydrates: 30g
- Fat: 12g
- Fiber: 6g
- Sugar: 2g
- Portion Size: 1 quesadilla

Vegan French Toast with Maple Syrup

Ingredients:

- 4 slices whole grain bread
- 1/2 cup unsweetened almond milk
- 1 tablespoon ground flaxseed
- 1 teaspoon vanilla extract
- 1/2 teaspoon ground cinnamon
- 1 tablespoon coconut oil (for cooking)
- Maple syrup for serving

Instructions:

1. In a shallow dish, whisk together almond milk, ground flaxseed, vanilla extract, and ground cinnamon.
2. Dip each slice of bread into the mixture, making sure to coat both sides evenly.
3. Heat coconut oil in a skillet over medium heat.
4. Cook the soaked bread slices for 3-4 minutes on each side until golden brown and crispy.
5. Serve hot with maple syrup drizzled on top.

Nutrition Information:
- Calories: 220
- Protein: 5g
- Carbohydrates: 30g
- Fat: 9g
- Fiber: 6g
- Sugar: 4g
- Portion Size: 2 slices

Blueberry Almond Smoothie

Ingredients:

- 1 cup frozen blueberries
- 1 ripe banana
- 1 tablespoon almond butter
- 1 cup almond milk
- 1 tablespoon chia seeds (optional)

Instructions:

1. In a blender, combine frozen blueberries, banana, almond butter, almond milk, and chia seeds if using.
2. Blend until smooth and creamy.
3. Pour into a glass and serve immediately as a refreshing and nutritious breakfast option.

Nutrition Information:

- Calories: 250
- Protein: 5g
- Carbohydrates: 35g
- Fat: 10g
- Fiber: 8g
- Sugar: 20g
- Portion Size: 1 serving

Chapter 3: Lunch Recipes

These recipes are carefully curated to provide a balance of protein, fiber, and essential nutrients while being mindful of your blood sugar levels. From hearty sandwiches to flavorful salads and satisfying bowls, each recipe offers a burst of flavor and nourishment without compromising on taste.

Chickpea Salad Sandwich with Whole Grain Bread

Ingredients:

- 1 can chickpeas, drained and rinsed
- 2 stalks celery, diced
- 1/4 cup red onion, finely chopped
- 2 tablespoons vegan mayonnaise
- 1 tablespoon Dijon mustard
- Salt and pepper to taste
- 4 slices whole grain bread
- Lettuce leaves and tomato slices for serving

Instructions:

1. In a bowl, mash the chickpeas with a fork until slightly chunky.

2. Add celery, red onion, vegan mayonnaise, Dijon mustard, salt, and pepper. Mix well to combine.

3. Divide the chickpea salad onto two slices of bread. Top with lettuce leaves and tomato slices, then cover with the remaining bread slices.

4. Slice the sandwiches in half and serve.

Nutrition Information (per serving):

- Calories: 320
- Protein: 12g
- Carbohydrates: 45g
- Fat: 10g
- Fiber: 10g
- Sugar: 6g
- Portion size: 1 sandwich

Lentil Soup with Spinach and Carrots

Ingredients:

- 1 cup green lentils, rinsed
- 4 cups vegetable broth
- 2 carrots, diced
- 2 cups fresh spinach
- 1 onion, diced
- 2 cloves garlic, minced
- 1 teaspoon cumin
- Salt and pepper to taste

Instructions:

1. In a large pot, sauté the onion and garlic until fragrant.
2. Add the lentils, vegetable broth, carrots, cumin, salt, and pepper. Bring to a boil, then reduce heat and simmer for 20-25 minutes until lentils are tender.
3. Stir in the spinach and cook for an additional 5 minutes until wilted.
4. Adjust seasoning if needed and serve hot.

Nutrition Information (per serving):

- Calories: 250
- Protein: 15g
- Carbohydrates: 40g
- Fat: 1g
- Fiber: 15g
- Sugar: 6g
- Portion size: 1 cup

Quinoa Salad with Roasted Vegetables

Ingredients:

- 1 cup quinoa, rinsed
- 2 cups mixed vegetables (such as bell peppers, zucchini, and cherry tomatoes), diced
- 2 tablespoons olive oil
- 2 tablespoons balsamic vinegar
- Salt and pepper to taste
- Fresh herbs (such as parsley or basil), chopped (optional)

Instructions:

1. Preheat the oven to 400°F (200°C).

2. In a bowl, toss the mixed vegetables with olive oil, balsamic vinegar, salt, and pepper.

3. Spread the vegetables on a baking sheet and roast for 20-25 minutes until tender and slightly caramelized.

4. Cook quinoa according to package instructions.

5. In a large bowl, combine cooked quinoa with roasted vegetables. Add fresh herbs if desired and toss to combine.

6. Serve warm or cold.

Nutrition Information (per serving):

- Calories: 280
- Protein: 8g
- Carbohydrates: 45g
- Fat: 8g
- Fiber: 6g
- Sugar: 4g
- Portion size: 1 cup

Vegan Caesar Salad with Tofu Croutons

Ingredients:

- 1 head romaine lettuce, chopped
- 1/2 cup cherry tomatoes, halved
- 1/4 cup vegan Caesar dressing
- 1/2 cup tofu, cubed
- 1 tablespoon olive oil
- 1 teaspoon garlic powder
- Salt and pepper to taste

Instructions:

1. Preheat the oven to 400°F (200°C).
2. Toss tofu cubes with olive oil, garlic powder, salt, and pepper.
3. Spread tofu on a baking sheet and bake for 20-25 minutes until crispy.
4. In a large bowl, combine chopped romaine lettuce and cherry tomatoes.
5. Drizzle vegan Caesar dressing over the salad and toss to coat.
6. Top with crispy tofu croutons and serve.

Nutrition Information (per serving):

- Calories: 220
- Protein: 10g
- Carbohydrates: 15g
- Fat: 15g
- Fiber: 5g
- Sugar: 3g
- Portion size: 1.5 cups

Stuffed Bell Peppers with Brown Rice and Black Beans

Ingredients:

- 4 bell peppers, halved and seeds removed
- 1 cup cooked brown rice
- 1 cup black beans, drained and rinsed
- 1 cup corn kernels
- 1/2 cup salsa
- 1 teaspoon cumin
- 1/2 teaspoon chili powder
- Salt and pepper to taste
- Vegan cheese for topping (optional)

Instructions:

1. Preheat the oven to 375°F (190°C).

2. In a bowl, mix together cooked brown rice, black beans, corn kernels, salsa, cumin, chili powder, salt, and pepper.

3. Stuff each bell pepper half with the rice and bean mixture.

4. Place stuffed peppers in a baking dish. Cover with foil and bake for 25-30 minutes until peppers are tender.

5. If using vegan cheese, sprinkle on top of the peppers during the last 5 minutes of baking.

6. Serve hot.

Nutrition Information (per serving):

- Calories: 280
- Protein: 10g
- Carbohydrates: 45g
- Fat: 5g
- Fiber: 10g
- Sugar: 6g
- Portion size: 1 stuffed pepper half

Greek Salad with Tofu Feta Cheese

Ingredients:

- 2 cups cherry tomatoes, halved
- 1 cucumber, diced
- 1/2 red onion, thinly sliced
- 1/4 cup Kalamata olives, pitted
- 1/4 cup fresh parsley, chopped
- 1 block firm tofu, pressed and cubed
- 2 tablespoons olive oil
- 2 tablespoons lemon juice
- 1 teaspoon dried oregano
- Salt and pepper to taste

Instructions:

1. In a large bowl, combine cherry tomatoes, cucumber, red onion, olives, and parsley.
2. In a separate bowl, whisk together olive oil, lemon juice, dried oregano, salt, and pepper to make the dressing.
3. Add tofu cubes to the dressing and toss to coat.
4. Add dressed tofu to the salad and toss gently to combine.

5. Serve chilled.

Nutrition Information (per serving):

- Calories: 240
- Protein: 15g
- Carbohydrates: 15g
- Fat: 15g
- Fiber: 5g
- Sugar: 6g
- Portion size: 1.5 cups

Mushroom and Spinach Quesadilla with Whole Wheat Tortillas

Ingredients:

- 4 whole wheat tortillas
- 2 cups mushrooms, sliced
- 2 cups fresh spinach
- 1/2 cup vegan cheese, shredded
- 1 tablespoon olive oil
- Salt and pepper to taste
- Salsa and guacamole for serving (optional)

Instructions:

1. In a skillet, heat olive oil over medium heat. Add mushrooms and cook until softened.
2. Add fresh spinach to the skillet and cook until wilted. Season with salt and pepper.
3. Place one tortilla in the skillet and sprinkle half of the vegan cheese over it.
4. Spoon the mushroom and spinach mixture over the cheese.
5. Sprinkle the remaining cheese on top and cover with another tortilla.
6. Cook until the bottom tortilla is golden brown, then flip and cook the other side.
7. Repeat with the remaining tortillas and filling.
8. Slice quesadillas into wedges and serve with salsa and guacamole if desired.

Nutrition Information (per serving):

- Calories: 320
- Protein: 12g
- Carbohydrates: 35g
- Fat: 15g

- Fiber: 8g
- Sugar: 2g
- Portion size: 1 quesadilla

Vegan BLT Wrap with Tempeh Bacon

Ingredients:

- 4 whole grain wraps
- 1 package tempeh, thinly sliced
- 4 lettuce leaves
- 2 tomatoes, sliced
- 1/4 cup vegan mayonnaise
- 2 tablespoons Dijon mustard
- Salt and pepper to taste

Instructions:

1. Heat a skillet over medium heat and add tempeh slices. Cook until crispy, about 3-4 minutes per side.
2. Spread vegan mayonnaise and Dijon mustard on each wrap.

3. Layer lettuce leaves, tomato slices, and cooked tempeh on each wrap.

4. Season with salt and pepper.

5. Roll up the wraps tightly and slice in half before serving.

Nutrition Information (per serving):

- Calories: 280
- Protein: 15g
- Carbohydrates: 30g
- Fat: 12g
- Fiber: 8g
- Sugar: 4g
- Portion size: 1 wrap

Thai Peanut Noodles with Tofu and Broccoli

Ingredients:

- 8 oz whole wheat spaghetti
- 1 block tofu, cubed
- 2 cups broccoli florets

- 1/4 cup peanut butter

- 2 tablespoons soy sauce

- 1 tablespoon maple syrup

- 1 tablespoon rice vinegar

- 1 teaspoon sesame oil

- 1 clove garlic, minced

- Crushed red pepper flakes (optional)

Instructions:

1. Cook spaghetti according to package instructions. Drain and set aside.

2. In a large skillet, heat sesame oil over medium heat. Add tofu cubes and cook until golden brown on all sides.

3. Add broccoli florets to the skillet and cook until tender-crisp.

4. In a small bowl, whisk together peanut butter, soy sauce, maple syrup, rice vinegar, garlic, and red pepper flakes if using.

5. Add cooked spaghetti to the skillet with tofu and broccoli. Pour the peanut sauce over the noodles and toss to coat.

6. Cook for an additional 2-3 minutes until heated
   through.
7. Serve hot.

Nutrition Information (per serving):

- Calories: 350
- Protein: 20g
- Carbohydrates: 45g
- Fat: 12g
- Fiber: 10g
- Sugar: 6g
- Portion size: 1.5 cups

Cauliflower Crust Pizza with Vegan Cheese

Ingredients:

- 1 small cauliflower head, grated
- 1 flaxseed egg (1 tablespoon ground flaxseed + 3 tablespoons water)
- 1/4 cup almond flour
- 1 teaspoon Italian seasoning

- Salt and pepper to taste

- 1/2 cup marinara sauce

- 1 cup vegan cheese, shredded

- Your favorite pizza toppings (such as mushrooms, bell peppers, and onions)

Instructions:

1. Preheat the oven to 425°F (220°C). Line a baking sheet with parchment paper.

2. In a bowl, mix grated cauliflower, flaxseed egg, almond flour, Italian seasoning, salt, and pepper until well combined.

3. Transfer the cauliflower mixture to the prepared baking sheet and spread it out into a circle, about 1/4 inch thick.

4. Bake the cauliflower crust for 20 minutes until golden brown and firm.

5. Remove from the oven and spread marinara sauce over the crust, leaving a border around the edges.

6. Sprinkle vegan cheese over the sauce and add your favorite pizza toppings.

7. Return the pizza to the oven and bake for an additional 10-12 minutes until the cheese is melted and bubbly.

8. Slice and serve hot.

Nutrition Information (per serving):

- Calories: 280
- Protein: 10g
- Carbohydrates: 25g
- Fat: 15g
- Fiber: 8g
- Sugar: 6g
- Portion size: 1 slice

Black Bean and Corn Salad with Lime Dressing

Ingredients:

- 2 cups black beans, cooked
- 1 cup corn kernels
- 1 red bell pepper, diced
- 1/4 cup red onion, finely chopped

- 1/4 cup fresh cilantro, chopped
- 2 tablespoons lime juice
- 1 tablespoon olive oil
- 1 teaspoon cumin
- Salt and pepper to taste
- Avocado slices for serving (optional)

Instructions:

1. In a large bowl, combine black beans, corn kernels, red bell pepper, red onion, and cilantro.
2. In a small bowl, whisk together lime juice, olive oil, cumin, salt, and pepper to make the dressing.
3. Pour the dressing over the salad and toss to coat evenly.
4. Chill the salad in the refrigerator for at least 30 minutes before serving.
5. Serve with avocado slices on top if desired.

Nutrition Information (per serving):

- Calories: 220
- Protein: 10g
- Carbohydrates: 30g

- Fat: 8g

- Fiber: 10g

- Sugar: 6g

- Portion size: 1 cup

Baked Falafel with Hummus and Pita Bread

Ingredients:

- 1 can chickpeas, drained and rinsed

- 2 cloves garlic, minced

- 1/4 cup fresh parsley, chopped

- 1 teaspoon ground cumin

- 1/2 teaspoon ground coriander

- 1/4 teaspoon cayenne pepper

- Salt and pepper to taste

- 2 tablespoons olive oil

- Hummus and whole wheat pita bread for serving

Instructions:

1. Preheat the oven to 375°F (190°C). Line a baking sheet with parchment paper.

2. In a food processor, combine chickpeas, garlic, parsley, cumin, coriander, cayenne pepper, salt, and pepper. Pulse until mixture is finely chopped and holds together when pressed.

3. Shape the mixture into small balls and flatten slightly to form patties.

4. Place the falafel patties on the prepared baking sheet and brush with olive oil.

5. Bake for 20-25 minutes, flipping halfway through, until falafel is golden brown and crispy.

6. Serve hot with hummus and whole wheat pita bread.

Nutrition Information (per serving):

- Calories: 220
- Protein: 10g
- Carbohydrates: 25g
- Fat: 10g
- Fiber: 8g
- Sugar: 4g
- Portion size: 3 falafel patties

Sweet Potato and Black Bean Burrito Bowl

Ingredients:

- 1 cup cooked brown rice
- 1 sweet potato, diced
- 1 cup black beans, cooked
- 1/2 cup corn kernels
- 1/4 cup salsa
- 1 avocado, sliced
- Fresh cilantro for garnish
- Lime wedges for serving

Instructions:

1. In a skillet, sauté sweet potato cubes until tender.
2. In a bowl, layer cooked brown rice, sautéed sweet potatoes, black beans, and corn kernels.
3. Top with salsa, avocado slices, and fresh cilantro.
4. Serve with lime wedges on the side for squeezing over the bowl.

Nutrition Information (per serving):

- Calories: 320

- Protein: 10g

- Carbohydrates: 45g

- Fat: 12g

- Fiber: 12g

- Sugar: 6g

- Portion size: 1.5 cups

Spinach and Mushroom Quiche with Tofu

Ingredients:

- 1 prepared whole wheat pie crust

- 1 block firm tofu, drained

- 2 cups fresh spinach, chopped

- 1 cup mushrooms, sliced

- 1/2 onion, diced

- 2 cloves garlic, minced

- 1/4 cup nutritional yeast

- 1 teaspoon turmeric

- Salt and pepper to taste

- Olive oil for cooking

Instructions:

1. Preheat the oven to 375°F (190°C).

2. Heat olive oil in a skillet over medium heat. Add onions and garlic, and cook until softened.

3. Add mushrooms and spinach to the skillet and cook until mushrooms are golden brown and spinach is wilted. Remove from heat and set aside.

4. In a food processor, blend tofu, nutritional yeast, turmeric, salt, and pepper until smooth and creamy.

5. Fold the cooked vegetables into the tofu mixture.

6. Pour the tofu mixture into the prepared pie crust and spread evenly.

7. Bake for 30-35 minutes until the quiche is set and the crust is golden brown.

8. Allow the quiche to cool for a few minutes before slicing and serving.

Nutrition Information (per serving):

- Calories: 280

- Protein: 12g

- Carbohydrates: 20g

- Fat: 15g

- Fiber: 5g
- Sugar: 3g
- Portion size: 1 slice

Vegan Sushi Rolls with Avocado and Cucumber

Ingredients:

- 2 nori seaweed sheets
- 1 cup sushi rice, cooked and seasoned with rice vinegar
- 1/2 avocado, thinly sliced
- 1/2 cucumber, julienned
- Soy sauce, for dipping
- Pickled ginger and wasabi, for serving (optional)

Instructions:

1. Place a nori seaweed sheet shiny side down on a bamboo sushi mat.
2. Spread a thin layer of sushi rice evenly over the nori sheet, leaving a 1-inch border at the top edge.

3. Arrange avocado slices and cucumber strips in the center of the rice.

4. Using the bamboo mat, roll the sushi tightly from the bottom, using gentle pressure to shape it into a cylinder.

5. Wet the top edge of the nori sheet with water to seal the roll.

6. Repeat with the remaining ingredients to make the second roll.

7. Slice each roll into 6-8 pieces using a sharp knife.

8. Serve the sushi rolls with soy sauce, pickled ginger, and wasabi on the side.

Nutrition Information (per serving, 1 roll):

- Calories: 150
- Protein: 3g
- Carbohydrates: 30g
- Fat: 2g
- Fiber: 3g
- Sugar: 1g
- Portion size: 1 roll

Chapter 4: Dinner Recipes

In this chapter, we've curated delicious dinner recipes that are not only vegan but also diabetes-friendly. Each recipe is carefully crafted to provide a balance of essential nutrients while keeping blood sugar levels in check.

Lentil Bolognese with Zucchini Noodles

Ingredients:

- 1 cup dried lentils
- 2 zucchinis, spiralized
- 1 onion, diced
- 2 cloves garlic, minced
- 1 can crushed tomatoes
- 1 tablespoon Italian seasoning
- Salt and pepper to taste

Instructions:

1. Cook lentils according to package instructions.

2. In a separate pan, sauté onion and garlic until translucent.

3. Add crushed tomatoes and Italian seasoning. Simmer for 10 minutes.

4. Stir in cooked lentils and season with salt and pepper.

5. Serve lentil Bolognese over zucchini noodles.

Nutrition Information:

- Calories: 250
- Protein: 15g
- Carbohydrates: 45g
- Fat: 1g
- Fiber: 12g
- Sugar: 10g
- Portion Size: 1 cup

Chickpea Curry with Brown Rice

Ingredients:

- 1 can chickpeas, drained and rinsed
- 1 onion, diced
- 2 cloves garlic, minced
- 1 tablespoon curry powder

- 1 can coconut milk

- 1 cup vegetable broth

- Cooked brown rice for serving

Instructions:

1. Sauté onion and garlic until softened.

2. Add chickpeas and curry powder. Cook for 2 minutes.

3. Pour in coconut milk and vegetable broth. Simmer for 15 minutes.

4. Serve chickpea curry over cooked brown rice.

Nutrition Information:

- Calories: 320

- Protein: 10g

- Carbohydrates: 40g

- Fat: 15g

- Fiber: 8g

- Sugar: 5g

- Portion Size: 1 cup curry with 1/2 cup brown rice

Vegan Chili with Quinoa and Kidney Beans

Ingredients:

- 1 cup quinoa, rinsed
- 1 onion, diced
- 2 cloves garlic, minced
- 1 bell pepper, diced
- 1 can diced tomatoes
- 1 can kidney beans, drained and rinsed
- 1 tablespoon chili powder
- Salt and pepper to taste

Instructions:

1. In a large pot, sauté onion, garlic, and bell pepper until softened.
2. Add diced tomatoes, quinoa, kidney beans, and chili powder.
3. Season with salt and pepper.
4. Simmer for 20 minutes or until quinoa is cooked.
5. Serve hot.

Nutrition Information:

- Calories: 280
- Protein: 12g
- Carbohydrates: 50g
- Fat: 3g
- Fiber: 10g
- Sugar: 8g
- Portion Size: 1 cup

Eggplant Parmesan with Marinara Sauce

Ingredients:

- 1 large eggplant, sliced
- 1 cup breadcrumbs (use whole wheat for a healthier option)
- 1 cup marinara sauce
- 1/2 cup vegan mozzarella cheese
- Fresh basil leaves for garnish

Instructions:

1. Preheat oven to 375°F (190°C).

2. Dip eggplant slices in breadcrumbs, ensuring they are evenly coated.

3. Place coated eggplant slices on a baking sheet and bake for 20 minutes, flipping halfway through.

4. In a baking dish, layer baked eggplant slices with marinara sauce and vegan mozzarella cheese.

5. Bake for an additional 15 minutes, until cheese is melted and bubbly.

6. Garnish with fresh basil leaves before serving.

Nutrition Information:

- Calories: 220
- Protein: 8g
- Carbohydrates: 30g
- Fat: 8g
- Fiber: 6g
- Sugar: 10g
- Portion Size: 1 serving (1/4 of the recipe)

Teriyaki Tofu Stir-Fry with Vegetables

Ingredients:

- 1 block extra firm tofu, pressed and cubed
- 2 cups mixed vegetables (such as bell peppers, broccoli, and snap peas)
- 1/4 cup teriyaki sauce (look for a low-sodium option)
- 1 tablespoon sesame oil
- Cooked brown rice for serving

Instructions:

1. Heat sesame oil in a large skillet over medium heat.
2. Add cubed tofu and stir-fry until golden brown.
3. Add mixed vegetables and continue to stir-fry until tender-crisp.
4. Pour teriyaki sauce over the tofu and vegetables. Stir to coat evenly.
5. Cook for an additional 2-3 minutes.
6. Serve hot over cooked brown rice.

Nutrition Information:

- Calories: 280

- Protein: 18g

- Carbohydrates: 30g

- Fat: 12g

- Fiber: 8g

- Sugar: 10g

- Portion Size: 1 cup stir-fry with 1/2 cup brown rice

Spaghetti Squash Pad Thai with Tofu

Ingredients:

- 1 spaghetti squash, halved and seeds removed

- 1 block firm tofu, pressed and cubed

- 2 tablespoons soy sauce (or tamari for gluten-free option)

- 1 tablespoon peanut butter

- 1 tablespoon lime juice

- 1 teaspoon sriracha sauce

- 2 cloves garlic, minced

- 1 cup bean sprouts

- Chopped peanuts and cilantro for garnish

Instructions:

1. Preheat oven to 400°F (200°C). Place spaghetti squash halves cut-side down on a baking sheet and roast for 30-40 minutes, until tender.
2. In a small bowl, whisk together soy sauce, peanut butter, lime juice, and sriracha sauce to make the sauce.
3. Heat a large skillet over medium heat and add cubed tofu. Cook until golden brown on all sides.
4. Add minced garlic to the skillet and cook for 1 minute.
5. Use a fork to scrape the cooked spaghetti squash into the skillet with the tofu.
6. Pour the sauce over the spaghetti squash and tofu. Stir to combine.
7. Add bean sprouts and cook for an additional 2-3 minutes.
8. Serve hot, garnished with chopped peanuts and cilantro.

Nutrition Information:

- Calories: 320

- Protein: 18g

- Carbohydrates: 30g

- Fat: 15g

- Fiber: 10g

- Sugar: 8g

- Portion Size: 1 cup

Stuffed Portobello Mushrooms with Couscous and Spinach

Ingredients:

- 4 large portobello mushrooms, stems removed

- 1 cup couscous, cooked

- 2 cups baby spinach, chopped

- 1/4 cup sun-dried tomatoes, chopped

- 1/4 cup vegan feta cheese, crumbled

- 2 tablespoons balsamic vinegar

- Salt and pepper to taste

Instructions:

1. Preheat oven to 375°F (190°C). Place portobello mushrooms on a baking sheet.

2. In a bowl, mix cooked couscous, chopped spinach, sun-dried tomatoes, vegan feta cheese, and balsamic vinegar. Season with salt and pepper.

3. Stuff each portobello mushroom with the couscous mixture.

4. Bake for 20-25 minutes, until mushrooms are tender.

5. Serve hot.

Nutrition Information:

- Calories: 200

- Protein: 10g

- Carbohydrates: 30g

- Fat: 5g

- Fiber: 6g

- Sugar: 5g

- Portion Size: 1 stuffed mushroom

Vegan Shepherd's Pie with Mashed Cauliflower

Ingredients:

- 1 head cauliflower, chopped into florets

- 2 tablespoons olive oil

- 1 onion, diced

- 2 cloves garlic, minced

- 2 carrots, diced

- 1 cup green peas

- 1 can lentils, drained and rinsed

- 1 cup vegetable broth

- 2 tablespoons tomato paste

- Salt and pepper to taste

Instructions:

1. Steam cauliflower florets until tender. Mash with a potato masher or blend in a food processor until smooth.

2. In a large skillet, heat olive oil over medium heat. Sauté onion, garlic, and carrots until softened.

3. Add green peas, lentils, vegetable broth, and tomato paste to the skillet. Season with salt and pepper. Simmer for 10 minutes.

4. Preheat oven to 375°F (190°C).

5. Transfer lentil mixture to a baking dish. Spread mashed cauliflower evenly over the top.

6. Bake for 20-25 minutes, until golden brown on top.

7. Serve hot.

Nutrition Information:

- Calories: 250
- Protein: 12g
- Carbohydrates: 35g
- Fat: 8g
- Fiber: 10g
- Sugar: 8g
- Portion Size: 1 cup

Mexican Quinoa Stuffed Peppers

Ingredients:

- 4 bell peppers, halved and seeds removed
- 1 cup quinoa, cooked
- 1 can black beans, drained and rinsed
- 1 cup corn kernels
- 1 cup diced tomatoes
- 1 teaspoon chili powder
- 1 teaspoon cumin
- 1/2 teaspoon paprika

- Salt and pepper to taste
- Fresh cilantro for garnish

Instructions:

1. Preheat oven to 375°F (190°C). Place bell pepper halves in a baking dish.
2. In a large bowl, mix together cooked quinoa, black beans, corn, diced tomatoes, chili powder, cumin, paprika, salt, and pepper.
3. Spoon quinoa mixture into each bell pepper half.
4. Cover the baking dish with foil and bake for 25-30 minutes, until peppers are tender.
5. Garnish with fresh cilantro before serving.

Nutrition Information:

- Calories: 280
- Protein: 10g
- Carbohydrates: 50g
- Fat: 2g
- Fiber: 12g
- Sugar: 8g
- Portion Size: 1 stuffed pepper half

Ratatouille with Polenta

Ingredients:

- 1 eggplant, diced
- 2 zucchinis, diced
- 1 yellow squash, diced
- 1 onion, diced
- 2 cloves garlic, minced
- 1 can diced tomatoes
- 1 tablespoon olive oil
- 1 teaspoon dried thyme
- 1 teaspoon dried basil
- Salt and pepper to taste
- Cooked polenta for serving

Instructions:

1. Heat olive oil in a large skillet over medium heat.
2. Sauté onion and garlic until softened.
3. Add diced eggplant, zucchini, and yellow squash to the skillet. Cook until vegetables are tender.
4. Stir in diced tomatoes, dried thyme, dried basil, salt, and pepper. Simmer for 10 minutes.
5. Serve ratatouille over cooked polenta.

Nutrition Information:

- Calories: 220
- Protein: 6g
- Carbohydrates: 40g
- Fat: 5g
- Fiber: 10g
- Sugar: 12g
- Portion Size: 1 cup ratatouille with 1/2 cup polenta

Jackfruit Tacos with Mango Salsa

Ingredients:

- 1 can young green jackfruit, drained and shredded
- 1 tablespoon olive oil
- 1 onion, diced
- 2 cloves garlic, minced
- 1 tablespoon taco seasoning
- 1 cup diced mango
- 1/2 cup diced red onion
- 1/4 cup chopped cilantro
- Juice of 1 lime
- Corn tortillas for serving

Instructions:

1. Heat olive oil in a skillet over medium heat. Add diced onion and minced garlic. Cook until softened.
2. Add shredded jackfruit and taco seasoning to the skillet. Cook for 5-7 minutes, until heated through and slightly caramelized.
3. In a separate bowl, combine diced mango, red onion, cilantro, and lime juice to make the salsa.
4. Warm corn tortillas in a dry skillet or microwave.
5. Assemble tacos by filling each tortilla with jackfruit mixture and topping with mango salsa.
6. Serve hot.

Nutrition Information:

- Calories: 220
- Protein: 5g
- Carbohydrates: 40g
- Fat: 6g
- Fiber: 8g
- Sugar: 12g
- Portion Size: 2 tacos

Butternut Squash Risotto with Sage

Ingredients:

- 1 butternut squash, peeled, seeded, and diced
- 1 onion, diced
- 2 cloves garlic, minced
- 1 cup Arborio rice
- 4 cups vegetable broth
- 1/2 cup dry white wine (optional)
- 2 tablespoons nutritional yeast
- Fresh sage leaves for garnish
- Salt and pepper to taste

Instructions:

1. In a large pot, heat vegetable broth over medium heat.
2. In a separate pan, sauté onion and garlic until softened.
3. Add Arborio rice to the pan and cook for 2-3 minutes, until translucent.
4. Pour in white wine (if using) and cook until absorbed.

5. Begin adding vegetable broth, 1/2 cup at a time, stirring frequently until absorbed before adding more.

6. Meanwhile, steam or roast diced butternut squash until tender.

7. When risotto is creamy and rice is cooked through, stir in cooked butternut squash and nutritional yeast.

8. Season with salt and pepper to taste.

9. Garnish with fresh sage leaves before serving.

Nutrition Information:

- Calories: 300
- Protein: 6g
- Carbohydrates: 50g
- Fat: 5g
- Fiber: 8g
- Sugar: 8g
- Portion Size: 1 cup

Cauliflower Alfredo Pasta with Peas and Mushrooms

Ingredients:

- 8 oz pasta of your choice (use whole wheat for a healthier option)
- 1 cauliflower head, chopped into florets
- 2 cloves garlic, minced
- 1 cup mushrooms, sliced
- 1 cup frozen peas
- 1 cup unsweetened almond milk
- 1/4 cup nutritional yeast
- Salt and pepper to taste
- Fresh parsley for garnish

Instructions:

1. Cook pasta according to package instructions. Drain and set aside.
2. Steam cauliflower florets until tender. Transfer to a blender.
3. In a skillet, sauté minced garlic and sliced mushrooms until softened.

4. Add frozen peas to the skillet and cook until heated through.

5. To the blender with cauliflower, add almond milk, nutritional yeast, salt, and pepper. Blend until smooth and creamy.

6. Pour cauliflower Alfredo sauce over cooked pasta. Add cooked mushrooms and peas. Stir to combine.

7. Serve hot, garnished with fresh parsley.

Nutrition Information:

- Calories: 320
- Protein: 12g
- Carbohydrates: 50g
- Fat: 6g
- Fiber: 10g
- Sugar: 6g
- Portion Size: 1 cup pasta

Veggie Stir-Fry with Quinoa

Ingredients:

- 1 cup quinoa, rinsed

- 2 cups mixed vegetables (such as bell peppers, broccoli, and carrots), sliced
- 1 onion, sliced
- 2 cloves garlic, minced
- 2 tablespoons low-sodium soy sauce (or tamari for gluten-free option)
- 1 tablespoon sesame oil
- 1 teaspoon ginger, grated
- Sesame seeds for garnish

Instructions:

1. Cook quinoa according to package instructions.
2. In a large skillet or wok, heat sesame oil over medium-high heat.
3. Add sliced onion and minced garlic. Stir-fry until fragrant.
4. Add mixed vegetables to the skillet and continue to stir-fry until tender-crisp.
5. Stir in cooked quinoa, low-sodium soy sauce, and grated ginger. Cook for an additional 2-3 minutes.
6. Serve hot, garnished with sesame seeds.

Nutrition Information:

- Calories: 280
- Protein: 10g
- Carbohydrates: 45g
- Fat: 8g
- Fiber: 10g
- Sugar: 6g
- Portion Size: 1 cup stir-fry with 1/2 cup quinoa

Vegan Gumbo with Okra and Brown Rice

Ingredients:

- 1 tablespoon olive oil
- 1 onion, diced
- 2 cloves garlic, minced
- 1 bell pepper, diced
- 2 stalks celery, diced
- 1 cup okra, sliced
- 1 can diced tomatoes
- 1 can kidney beans, drained and rinsed
- 4 cups vegetable broth

- 1 tablespoon Cajun seasoning

- 1/4 teaspoon cayenne pepper (adjust to taste)

- Cooked brown rice for serving

- Fresh parsley for garnish

Instructions:

1. In a large pot, heat olive oil over medium heat. Add diced onion, minced garlic, diced bell pepper, and diced celery. Sauté until softened.

2. Add sliced okra to the pot and cook for 5 minutes, stirring occasionally.

3. Stir in diced tomatoes, drained kidney beans, vegetable broth, Cajun seasoning, and cayenne pepper.

4. Bring the mixture to a boil, then reduce heat and simmer for 20-25 minutes.

5. Serve hot over cooked brown rice.

6. Garnish with fresh parsley before serving.

Nutrition Information:

- Calories: 280

- Protein: 10g

- Carbohydrates: 45g

- Fat: 6g

- Fiber: 12g

- Sugar: 8g

- Portion Size: 1 cup gumbo with 1/2 cup brown rice

Chapter 5: Snacks and Appetizers

In this chapter, we'll explore delightful vegan options that are perfect for nibbling on solo or sharing with friends. From creamy dips to crunchy bites, these recipes are not only delicious but also packed with nutrients to keep you energized throughout the day.

Guacamole with Baked Tortilla Chips

Ingredients:

- 2 ripe avocados
- 1 tomato, diced
- 1/4 cup red onion, finely chopped
- 1 jalapeño, seeded and minced
- 1 lime, juiced
- Salt and pepper to taste
- Baked tortilla chips, for serving

Instructions:

1. Mash the avocados in a bowl until smooth.

2. Stir in the diced tomato, chopped red onion, minced jalapeño, and lime juice.

3. Season with salt and pepper to taste.

4. Serve with baked tortilla chips.

Nutrition Information:

- Calories: 180
- Protein: 3g
- Carbohydrates: 15g
- Fat: 13g
- Fiber: 7g
- Sugar: 2g
- Portion size: 1/4 cup guacamole with 10 tortilla chips

Hummus with Carrot Sticks and Celery

Ingredients:

- 1 can (15 ounces) chickpeas, drained and rinsed
- 2 cloves garlic, minced
- 2 tablespoons tahini
- 2 tablespoons lemon juice

- 2 tablespoons olive oil

- Salt to taste

- Carrot sticks and celery, for dipping

Instructions:

1. In a food processor, combine the chickpeas, minced garlic, tahini, lemon juice, and olive oil.

2. Blend until smooth, adding water as needed to reach desired consistency.

3. Season with salt to taste.

4. Serve with carrot sticks and celery for dipping.

Nutrition Information:

- Calories: 120

- Protein: 4g

- Carbohydrates: 10g

- Fat: 7g

- Fiber: 3g

- Sugar: 1g

- Portion size: 1/4 cup hummus with 1 cup carrot and celery sticks

Edamame with Sea Salt

Ingredients:

- 2 cups frozen edamame, thawed
- Sea salt to taste

Instructions:

1. Bring a pot of water to a boil.
2. Add the edamame and cook for 3-5 minutes, or until tender.
3. Drain the edamame and sprinkle with sea salt.
4. Serve warm or chilled.

Nutrition Information:

- Calories: 120
- Protein: 11g
- Carbohydrates: 9g
- Fat: 4g
- Fiber: 6g
- Sugar: 2g
- Portion size: 1 cup edamame

Roasted Chickpeas with Spices

Ingredients:

- 1 can (15 ounces) chickpeas, drained and rinsed
- 1 tablespoon olive oil
- 1 teaspoon paprika
- 1/2 teaspoon cumin
- 1/2 teaspoon garlic powder
- Salt and pepper to taste

Instructions:

1. Preheat the oven to 400°F (200°C).
2. Pat the chickpeas dry with a paper towel and transfer them to a baking sheet.
3. Drizzle with olive oil and sprinkle with paprika, cumin, garlic powder, salt, and pepper.
4. Toss to coat evenly.
5. Roast in the oven for 25-30 minutes, stirring halfway through, until crispy.
6. Let cool before serving.

Nutrition Information:

- Calories: 150

- Protein: 6g

- Carbohydrates: 20g

- Fat: 5g

- Fiber: 6g

- Sugar: 1g

- Portion size: 1/4 cup roasted chickpeas

Sliced Cucumber with Lemon and Tajin

Ingredients:

- 2 cucumbers, sliced

- 1 lemon, juiced

- Tajin seasoning to taste

Instructions:

1. Arrange the cucumber slices on a serving platter.

2. Drizzle with freshly squeezed lemon juice.

3. Sprinkle with Tajin seasoning to taste.

4. Serve immediately.

Nutrition Information:

- Calories: 15
- Protein: 1g
- Carbohydrates: 3g
- Fat: 0g
- Fiber: 1g
- Sugar: 1g
- Portion size: 1 cup sliced cucumber

Vegan Cheese and Crackers

Ingredients:

- Vegan cheese of your choice
- Whole grain crackers

Instructions:

1. Arrange the vegan cheese and crackers on a serving platter.
2. Serve immediately.

Nutrition Information:

- Calories: Varies depending on cheese and crackers
- Protein: Varies

- Carbohydrates: Varies

- Fat: Varies

- Fiber: Varies

- Sugar: Varies

- Portion size: Varies

Trail Mix with Nuts and Dried Fruit

Ingredients:

- 1 cup mixed nuts (almonds, cashews, walnuts)

- 1/2 cup dried fruit (raisins, cranberries, apricots)

- 1/4 cup dark chocolate chips (optional)

Instructions:

1. In a bowl, combine the mixed nuts, dried fruit, and dark chocolate chips (if using).

2. Mix well to combine.

3. Portion into individual servings or store in an airtight container for later.

Nutrition Information:

- Calories: 200

- Protein: 5g

- Carbohydrates: 20g

- Fat: 12g

- Fiber: 4g

- Sugar: 10g

- Portion size: 1/4 cup trail mix

Avocado Salsa with Whole Grain Crackers

Ingredients:

- 2 ripe avocados, diced

- 1 tomato, diced

- 1/4 cup red onion, finely chopped

- 1 jalapeño, seeded and minced

- 1 lime, juiced

- Salt and pepper to taste

- Whole grain crackers, for serving

Instructions:

1. In a bowl, combine the diced avocados, tomato, red onion, minced jalapeño, and lime juice.

2. Season with salt and pepper to taste.

3. Gently toss to combine.

4. Serve with whole grain crackers.

Nutrition Information:

- Calories: 150
- Protein: 2g
- Carbohydrates: 10g
- Fat: 12g
- Fiber: 6g
- Sugar: 2g
- Portion size: 1/4 cup avocado salsa with 10 whole grain crackers

Stuffed Mini Bell Peppers with Vegan Cream Cheese

Ingredients:

- 12 mini bell peppers
- 1/2 cup vegan cream cheese
- 2 tablespoons chopped fresh herbs (such as parsley or chives)

Instructions:

1. Slice the tops off the mini bell peppers and remove the seeds.
2. In a bowl, mix together the vegan cream cheese and chopped fresh herbs.
3. Stuff each mini bell pepper with the cream cheese mixture.
4. Arrange on a serving platter and serve immediately.

Nutrition Information:

- Calories: 70
- Protein: 2g
- Carbohydrates: 5g
- Fat: 5g
- Fiber: 1g
- Sugar: 3g
- Portion size: 3 stuffed mini bell peppers

Caprese Skewers with Cherry Tomatoes and Basil

Ingredients:

- Cherry tomatoes
- Fresh basil leaves
- Vegan mozzarella-style cheese, cubed
- Balsamic glaze (optional)

Instructions:

1. Thread a cherry tomato, a basil leaf, and a cube of vegan mozzarella onto each skewer.
2. Repeat until all skewers are assembled.
3. Drizzle with balsamic glaze, if desired, before serving.

Nutrition Information:

- Calories: 30
- Protein: 2g
- Carbohydrates: 2g
- Fat: 1g
- Fiber: 1g
- Sugar: 1g
- Portion size: 1 skewer

Baked Sweet Potato Fries with Chipotle Aioli

Ingredients:

- 2 large sweet potatoes, cut into fries
- 1 tablespoon olive oil
- Salt and pepper to taste
- 1/4 cup vegan mayonnaise
- 1 chipotle pepper in adobo sauce, minced
- 1 teaspoon adobo sauce
- 1 clove garlic, minced
- 1 tablespoon lime juice

Instructions:

1. Preheat the oven to 425°F (220°C).
2. Toss the sweet potato fries with olive oil, salt, and pepper on a baking sheet.
3. Spread the fries in a single layer and bake for 20-25 minutes, flipping halfway through, until crispy.
4. Meanwhile, prepare the chipotle aioli by mixing together the vegan mayonnaise, minced chipotle pepper, adobo sauce, garlic, and lime juice.

5. Serve the baked sweet potato fries with the chipotle aioli for dipping.

Nutrition Information:

- Calories: 150
- Protein: 2g
- Carbohydrates: 20g
- Fat: 7g
- Fiber: 3g
- Sugar: 5g
- Portion size: 1/2 cup baked sweet potato fries with 2 tablespoons chipotle aioli

Spinach Artichoke Dip with Whole Wheat Pita Chips

Ingredients:

- 1 can (14 ounces) artichoke hearts, drained and chopped
- 1 cup frozen chopped spinach, thawed and drained
- 1 cup vegan cream cheese
- 1/2 cup vegan mayonnaise

- 1/4 cup nutritional yeast

- 2 cloves garlic, minced

- Salt and pepper to taste

- Whole wheat pita bread, cut into triangles

Instructions:

1. Preheat the oven to 350°F (175°C).

2. In a bowl, mix together the chopped artichoke hearts, chopped spinach, vegan cream cheese, vegan mayonnaise, nutritional yeast, minced garlic, salt, and pepper.

3. Transfer the mixture to a baking dish and spread it out evenly.

4. Bake for 25-30 minutes, until bubbly and golden brown on top.

5. While the dip is baking, arrange the whole wheat pita triangles on a baking sheet and bake for 8-10 minutes, until crisp.

6. Serve the spinach artichoke dip warm with the whole wheat pita chips.

Nutrition Information:

- Calories: 120
- Protein: 4g
- Carbohydrates: 10g
- Fat: 7g
- Fiber: 3g
- Sugar: 1g
- Portion size: 1/4 cup dip with 6 whole wheat pita chips

Vegan Spring Rolls with Peanut Dipping Sauce

Ingredients:

- Rice paper wrappers
- Thinly sliced vegetables (such as carrots, cucumbers, bell peppers, and lettuce)
- Cooked rice noodles
- Fresh herbs (such as cilantro, mint, and basil)
- Peanut dipping sauce (store-bought or homemade)

Instructions:

1. Prepare a shallow dish of warm water.
2. Dip one rice paper wrapper into the water until softened, then lay it flat on a clean surface.
3. Arrange a small handful of rice noodles and sliced vegetables on the lower third of the wrapper.
4. Top with fresh herbs.
5. Fold the bottom of the wrapper over the filling, then fold in the sides, and roll tightly.
6. Repeat with the remaining wrappers and filling ingredients.
7. Serve the spring rolls with peanut dipping sauce.

Nutrition Information:

- Calories: 80 (per spring roll)
- Protein: 3g
- Carbohydrates: 15g
- Fat: 1g
- Fiber: 2g
- Sugar: 2g
- Portion size: 1 spring roll with dipping sauce

Roasted Vegetable Platter with Balsamic Glaze

Ingredients:

- Assorted vegetables (such as bell peppers, zucchini, eggplant, cherry tomatoes, and mushrooms)
- Olive oil
- Salt and pepper to taste
- Balsamic glaze

Instructions:

1. Preheat the oven to 425°F (220°C).
2. Cut the vegetables into bite-sized pieces and place them on a baking sheet.
3. Drizzle with olive oil and season with salt and pepper.
4. Roast in the oven for 20-25 minutes, or until tender and caramelized.
5. Arrange the roasted vegetables on a platter and drizzle with balsamic glaze before serving.

Nutrition Information:

- Calories: Varies depending on vegetables

- Protein: Varies
- Carbohydrates: Varies
- Fat: Varies
- Fiber: Varies
- Sugar: Varies
- Portion size: Varies

Seaweed Snacks with Wasabi Peas

Ingredients:

- Seaweed snacks
- Wasabi peas

Instructions:

1. Open the seaweed snacks and wasabi peas packages.
2. Serve together as a crunchy and savory snack combination.

Nutrition Information:

- Calories: 50 (per seaweed snack pack)
- Protein: 1g
- Carbohydrates: 1g
- Fat: 2g

- Fiber: 1g

- Sugar: 0g

- Portion size: 1 seaweed snack pack with a small handful of wasabi peas

Chapter 6: Desserts

In this chapter, you'll discover a collection of vegan desserts designed to satisfy your sweet cravings while aligning with your dietary needs. So, let's dive into the world of guilt-free indulgence and treat yourself to these delectable vegan desserts!

Vegan Chocolate Avocado Mousse

Ingredients:

- 2 ripe avocados
- 1/4 cup cocoa powder
- 1/4 cup maple syrup
- 1 tsp vanilla extract
- Pinch of salt

Instructions:

1. Scoop out the flesh of the avocados and place them in a blender or food processor.
2. Add cocoa powder, maple syrup, vanilla extract, and a pinch of salt.

3. Blend until smooth and creamy.

4. Divide the mousse into serving dishes and refrigerate for at least 1 hour before serving.

Nutrition Information (per serving):

- Calories: 200
- Protein: 3g
- Carbohydrates: 20g
- Fat: 15g
- Fiber: 8g
- Sugar: 10g
- Portion Size: 1/2 cup

Banana Ice Cream with Almond Butter Drizzle

Ingredients:

- 4 ripe bananas, frozen
- 2 tbsp almond butter

Instructions:

1. Peel the bananas and cut them into chunks.

2. Place the banana chunks in a blender or food processor.
3. Blend until smooth and creamy, resembling ice cream.
4. Drizzle almond butter over the banana ice cream before serving.

Nutrition Information (per serving):

- Calories: 180
- Protein: 2g
- Carbohydrates: 30g
- Fat: 7g
- Fiber: 4g
- Sugar: 15g
- Portion Size: 1 cup

Berry Crisp with Oat Topping

Ingredients:

- 4 cups mixed berries (such as strawberries, blueberries, and raspberries)
- 1/4 cup maple syrup
- 1 tbsp cornstarch

- 1 cup rolled oats
- 1/4 cup almond flour
- 1/4 cup coconut oil, melted
- 1/4 cup chopped nuts (such as almonds or walnuts)
- 1 tsp cinnamon

Instructions:

1. Preheat the oven to 350°F (175°C).
2. In a mixing bowl, combine the mixed berries, maple syrup, and cornstarch. Mix until the berries are coated evenly.
3. Transfer the berry mixture into a baking dish.
4. In a separate bowl, mix together rolled oats, almond flour, melted coconut oil, chopped nuts, and cinnamon until well combined.
5. Sprinkle the oat topping evenly over the berry mixture.
6. Bake in the preheated oven for 30-35 minutes, or until the topping is golden brown and the berries are bubbling.
7. Allow to cool slightly before serving.

Nutrition Information (per serving):

- Calories: 250
- Protein: 4g
- Carbohydrates: 35g
- Fat: 11g
- Fiber: 6g
- Sugar: 18g
- Portion Size: 1/2 cup

Vegan Cheesecake with Strawberry Sauce

Ingredients:

- 1 1/2 cups raw cashews, soaked overnight
- 1/2 cup coconut cream
- 1/4 cup lemon juice
- 1/4 cup maple syrup
- 1 tsp vanilla extract
- 1/4 cup coconut oil, melted
- 1 cup strawberries, sliced
- 2 tbsp maple syrup
- 1 tbsp lemon juice

Instructions:

1. In a food processor, blend soaked cashews, coconut cream, lemon juice, maple syrup, vanilla extract, and melted coconut oil until smooth and creamy.
2. Pour the mixture into a springform pan and smooth the top with a spatula.
3. Place the pan in the freezer for 4-6 hours, or until firm.
4. In a small saucepan, combine sliced strawberries, maple syrup, and lemon juice. Cook over medium heat until the strawberries are soft and syrupy.
5. Allow the strawberry sauce to cool before serving.
6. Remove the cheesecake from the freezer and let it sit at room temperature for 10-15 minutes before slicing.
7. Serve each slice with a drizzle of strawberry sauce.

Nutrition Information (per serving):

- Calories: 300
- Protein: 6g
- Carbohydrates: 25g
- Fat: 20g

- Fiber: 3g
- Sugar: 15g
- Portion Size: 1 slice

Apple Cinnamon Energy Bites

Ingredients:

- 1 cup rolled oats
- 1/2 cup unsweetened applesauce
- 1/4 cup almond butter
- 2 tbsp maple syrup
- 1 tsp cinnamon
- 1/4 cup chopped dried apples
- 1/4 cup chopped almonds

Instructions:

1. In a mixing bowl, combine rolled oats, applesauce, almond butter, maple syrup, and cinnamon until well mixed.

2. Fold in chopped dried apples and almonds until evenly distributed.

3. Roll the mixture into bite-sized balls using your hands.

4. Place the energy bites on a baking sheet lined with parchment paper.

5. Refrigerate for at least 30 minutes before serving.

Nutrition Information (per serving):

- Calories: 120
- Protein: 3g
- Carbohydrates: 15g
- Fat: 6g
- Fiber: 2g
- Sugar: 6g
- Portion Size: 2 bites

Pumpkin Spice Oat Bars

Ingredients:

- 2 cups rolled oats
- 1/2 cup pumpkin puree
- 1/4 cup maple syrup
- 1/4 cup almond butter
- 1 tsp pumpkin pie spice
- 1/4 cup chopped pecans

Instructions:

1. Preheat the oven to 350°F (175°C). Grease a baking dish with coconut oil.
2. In a mixing bowl, combine rolled oats, pumpkin puree, maple syrup, almond butter, and pumpkin pie spice. Mix until well combined.
3. Fold in chopped pecans.
4. Press the mixture into the prepared baking dish, spreading it out evenly.
5. Bake for 25-30 minutes, or until the edges are golden brown.
6. Allow to cool before cutting into bars.

Nutrition Information (per serving):

- Calories: 150
- Protein: 4g
- Carbohydrates: 20g
- Fat: 7g
- Fiber: 3g
- Sugar: 6g
- Portion Size: 1 bar

Chocolate Chip Chickpea Cookies

Ingredients:

- 1 can (15 oz) chickpeas, drained and rinsed
- 1/2 cup almond butter
- 1/4 cup maple syrup
- 1 tsp vanilla extract
- 1/2 tsp baking powder
- Pinch of salt
- 1/4 cup vegan chocolate chips

Instructions:

1. Preheat the oven to 350°F (175°C). Line a baking sheet with parchment paper.
2. In a food processor, blend chickpeas, almond butter, maple syrup, vanilla extract, baking powder, and salt until smooth.
3. Transfer the mixture to a mixing bowl and fold in the vegan chocolate chips.
4. Drop spoonfuls of dough onto the prepared baking sheet, spacing them apart.
5. Flatten each cookie slightly with the back of a spoon.

6. Bake for 12-15 minutes, or until the edges are golden brown.

7. Allow to cool on the baking sheet for 5 minutes before transferring to a wire rack to cool completely.

Nutrition Information (per serving, based on 2 cookies):

- Calories: 150
- Protein: 5g
- Carbohydrates: 18g
- Fat: 7g
- Fiber: 4g
- Sugar: 8g
- Portion Size: 2 cookies

Coconut Mango Sorbet

Ingredients:

- 2 cups frozen mango chunks
- 1/2 cup coconut milk
- 2 tbsp maple syrup (optional, adjust to taste)

Instructions:

1. In a blender or food processor, combine frozen mango chunks, coconut milk, and maple syrup (if using).
2. Blend until smooth and creamy, scraping down the sides as needed.
3. Transfer the sorbet to a container and freeze for at least 2 hours before serving.
4. Scoop into bowls and garnish with fresh mango slices or shredded coconut if desired.

Nutrition Information (per serving):

- Calories: 120
- Protein: 1g
- Carbohydrates: 25g
- Fat: 3g
- Fiber: 3g
- Sugar: 20g
- Portion Size: 1/2 cup

Lemon Poppy Seed Muffins

Ingredients:

- 1 1/2 cups all-purpose flour
- 1/2 cup almond flour
- 1/2 cup coconut sugar
- 2 tsp baking powder
- 1/4 tsp salt
- 1/4 cup melted coconut oil
- 1 cup almond milk
- Zest of 1 lemon
- 2 tbsp lemon juice
- 1 tbsp poppy seeds

Instructions:

1. Preheat the oven to 375°F (190°C). Line a muffin tin with paper liners.

2. In a large mixing bowl, combine all-purpose flour, almond flour, coconut sugar, baking powder, and salt.

3. In a separate bowl, whisk together melted coconut oil, almond milk, lemon zest, and lemon juice.

4. Pour the wet ingredients into the dry ingredients and stir until just combined.

5. Fold in poppy seeds until evenly distributed throughout the batter.

6. Spoon the batter into the prepared muffin tin, filling each cup about 3/4 full.

7. Bake for 18-20 minutes, or until a toothpick inserted into the center comes out clean.

8. Allow the muffins to cool in the tin for 5 minutes before transferring to a wire rack to cool completely.

Nutrition Information (per serving, based on 1 muffin):

- Calories: 180
- Protein: 3g
- Carbohydrates: 22g
- Fat: 9g
- Fiber: 2g
- Sugar: 9g
- Portion Size: 1 muffin

Peanut Butter Banana Cookies

Ingredients:

- 2 ripe bananas, mashed
- 1/2 cup peanut butter
- 1/4 cup coconut sugar
- 1 tsp vanilla extract
- 1 1/4 cups rolled oats
- 1/4 cup chopped peanuts (optional)

Instructions:

1. Preheat the oven to 350°F (175°C). Line a baking sheet with parchment paper.
2. In a mixing bowl, combine mashed bananas, peanut butter, coconut sugar, and vanilla extract until smooth.
3. Stir in rolled oats and chopped peanuts (if using) until well combined.
4. Drop spoonfuls of dough onto the prepared baking sheet, spacing them apart.
5. Flatten each cookie slightly with the back of a spoon.
6. Bake for 12-15 minutes, or until the edges are golden brown.

7. Allow to cool on the baking sheet for 5 minutes before transferring to a wire rack to cool completely.

Nutrition Information (per serving, based on 2 cookies):

- Calories: 200
- Protein: 6g
- Carbohydrates: 22g
- Fat: 10g
- Fiber: 3g
- Sugar: 9g
- Portion Size: 2 cookies

Raspberry Chia Seed Jam Bars

Ingredients:

- 1 1/2 cups rolled oats
- 1/2 cup almond flour
- 1/4 cup coconut oil, melted
- 1/4 cup maple syrup
- 1/2 cup raspberry chia seed jam (store-bought or homemade)

Instructions:

1. Preheat the oven to 350°F (175°C). Grease a baking dish with coconut oil or line it with parchment paper.

2. In a mixing bowl, combine rolled oats, almond flour, melted coconut oil, and maple syrup. Mix until well combined and the mixture resembles coarse crumbs.

3. Press half of the oat mixture into the bottom of the prepared baking dish, forming an even layer.

4. Spread raspberry chia seed jam evenly over the oat layer.

5. Sprinkle the remaining oat mixture over the jam layer, pressing down lightly.

6. Bake for 25-30 minutes, or until the top is golden brown.

7. Allow to cool completely before cutting into bars.

Nutrition Information (per serving, based on 1 bar):

- Calories: 180
- Protein: 3g
- Carbohydrates: 22g
- Fat: 9g
- Fiber: 3g

- Sugar: 9g
- Portion Size: 1 bar

Almond Butter Cups with Dark Chocolate

Ingredients:

- 1/2 cup almond butter
- 2 tbsp maple syrup
- 1/4 tsp vanilla extract
- 1 cup dark chocolate chips
- Sea salt flakes (optional, for topping)

Instructions:

1. Line a mini muffin tin with paper liners.
2. In a mixing bowl, combine almond butter, maple syrup, and vanilla extract until smooth.
3. Melt dark chocolate chips in a microwave-safe bowl in 30-second intervals, stirring in between, until smooth.

4. Spoon a small amount of melted chocolate into the bottom of each muffin liner, spreading it out to cover the bottom.

5. Place a small dollop of almond butter mixture on top of the chocolate layer in each liner.

6. Cover the almond butter layer with more melted chocolate, smoothing it out with the back of a spoon.

7. Sprinkle sea salt flakes on top if desired.

8. Refrigerate for at least 30 minutes, or until the almond butter cups are set.

9. Store in the refrigerator until ready to serve.

Nutrition Information (per serving, based on 1 almond butter cup):

- Calories: 150
- Protein: 3g
- Carbohydrates: 12g
- Fat: 10g
- Fiber: 2g
- Sugar: 7g
- Portion Size: 1 almond butter cup

Blueberry Coconut Popsicles

Ingredients:

- 1 1/2 cups fresh or frozen blueberries
- 1 cup coconut milk
- 2 tbsp maple syrup
- 1 tsp vanilla extract

Instructions:

1. In a blender, combine blueberries, coconut milk, maple syrup, and vanilla extract.
2. Blend until smooth and well combined.
3. Pour the mixture into popsicle molds.
4. Insert popsicle sticks into the molds.
5. Freeze for at least 4 hours, or until the popsicles are completely frozen.
6. To remove the popsicles from the molds, run warm water over the outside of the molds for a few seconds.
7. Serve immediately and enjoy the refreshing treat!

Nutrition Information (per serving, based on 1 popsicle):

- Calories: 70

- Protein: 1g

- Carbohydrates: 10g

- Fat: 4g

- Fiber: 1g

- Sugar: 7g

- Portion Size: 1 popsicle

Carrot Cake Energy Balls

Ingredients:

- 1 cup rolled oats

- 1/2 cup shredded carrots

- 1/4 cup chopped walnuts

- 1/4 cup raisins

- 2 tbsp maple syrup

- 1 tbsp almond butter

- 1/2 tsp cinnamon

- Pinch of nutmeg

Instructions:

1. In a food processor, combine rolled oats, shredded carrots, chopped walnuts, raisins, maple syrup, almond butter, cinnamon, and nutmeg.

2. Pulse until the mixture comes together and forms a dough-like consistency.

3. Roll the mixture into balls, using about 1 tablespoon of mixture for each ball.

4. Place the energy balls on a baking sheet lined with parchment paper.

5. Refrigerate for at least 30 minutes before serving.

6. Store the energy balls in an airtight container in the refrigerator for up to one week.

Nutrition Information (per serving, based on 2 energy balls):

- Calories: 100
- Protein: 2g
- Carbohydrates: 15g
- Fat: 4g
- Fiber: 2g
- Sugar: 6g
- Portion Size: 2 energy balls

Vegan Rice Pudding with Cinnamon

Ingredients:

- 1 cup cooked white rice

- 2 cups coconut milk
- 1/4 cup maple syrup
- 1 tsp vanilla extract
- 1/2 tsp ground cinnamon
- Pinch of salt
- Optional toppings: sliced almonds, raisins, fresh fruit

Instructions:

1. In a saucepan, combine cooked white rice, coconut milk, maple syrup, vanilla extract, ground cinnamon, and a pinch of salt.
2. Bring the mixture to a simmer over medium heat, stirring occasionally.
3. Reduce the heat to low and continue to simmer for 20-25 minutes, or until the rice pudding thickens.
4. Remove from heat and let cool slightly.
5. Serve warm or chilled, topped with sliced almonds, raisins, or fresh fruit if desired.
6. Enjoy this comforting vegan rice pudding as a delicious dessert or snack!

Nutrition Information (per serving):

- Calories: 200
- Protein: 2g
- Carbohydrates: 25g
- Fat: 10g
- Fiber: 1g
- Sugar: 10g
- Portion Size: 1/2 cup

Chapter 7: Smoothies

In this chapter, you'll discover smoothie recipes designed to tantalize your taste buds while nourishing your body. Whether you're in need of a quick breakfast on-the-go, a post-workout refuel, or a refreshing snack, these smoothies have got you covered.

Green Detox Smoothie with Kale and Pineapple

Ingredients:

- 1 cup chopped kale
- 1 cup fresh pineapple chunks
- 1 ripe banana
- 1/2 cup coconut water
- 1 tablespoon fresh lemon juice

Instructions:

1. Add all ingredients to a blender.
2. Blend until smooth and creamy.
3. Serve immediately.

Nutrition Information:

- Calories: 150
- Protein: 3g
- Carbohydrates: 35g
- Fat: 1g
- Fiber: 5g
- Sugar: 20g
- Portion size: 1 smoothie

Strawberry Banana Smoothie with Spinach

Ingredients:

- 1 cup fresh spinach
- 1 cup frozen strawberries
- 1 ripe banana
- 1/2 cup almond milk
- 1 tablespoon honey or maple syrup (optional)

Instructions:

1. Combine all ingredients in a blender.
2. Blend until smooth and creamy.

3. Pour into glasses and enjoy.

Nutrition Information:
- Calories: 140
- Protein: 2g
- Carbohydrates: 32g
- Fat: 1g
- Fiber: 5g
- Sugar: 20g
- Portion size: 1 smoothie

Mango Coconut Smoothie with Turmeric

Ingredients:
- 1 cup frozen mango chunks
- 1/2 cup coconut milk
- 1/2 cup coconut water
- 1 teaspoon ground turmeric
- 1 tablespoon honey or agave syrup (optional)

Instructions:

1. Place all ingredients in a blender.

2. Blend until smooth and creamy.

3. Pour into glasses and serve immediately.

Nutrition Information:

- Calories: 180

- Protein: 2g

- Carbohydrates: 30g

- Fat: 7g

- Fiber: 3g

- Sugar: 25g

- Portion size: 1 smoothie

Blueberry Almond Butter Smoothie

Ingredients:

- 1 cup frozen blueberries

- 1 tablespoon almond butter

- 1/2 cup almond milk

- 1/2 cup plain Greek yogurt

- 1 tablespoon honey or maple syrup (optional)

Instructions:

1. Combine all ingredients in a blender.
2. Blend until smooth and creamy.
3. Pour into glasses and serve immediately.

Nutrition Information:

- Calories: 200
- Protein: 10g
- Carbohydrates: 30g
- Fat: 6g
- Fiber: 5g
- Sugar: 20g
- Portion size: 1 smoothie

Chocolate Peanut Butter Protein Smoothie

Ingredients:

- 1 ripe banana
- 2 tablespoons cocoa powder
- 2 tablespoons peanut butter
- 1 cup unsweetened almond milk

- 1 scoop chocolate protein powder

Instructions:

1. Combine all ingredients in a blender.
2. Blend until smooth and creamy.
3. Serve immediately.

Nutrition Information:

- Calories: 320
- Protein: 20g
- Carbohydrates: 30g
- Fat: 14g
- Fiber: 8g
- Sugar: 12g
- Portion size: 1 smoothie

Raspberry Oatmeal Smoothie

Ingredients:

- 1/2 cup rolled oats
- 1 cup frozen raspberries
- 1 ripe banana
- 1 cup almond milk

- 1 tablespoon honey or maple syrup (optional)

Instructions:

1. Add all ingredients to a blender.

2. Blend until smooth and creamy.

3. Pour into glasses and enjoy.

Nutrition Information:

- Calories: 250

- Protein: 6g

- Carbohydrates: 45g

- Fat: 5g

- Fiber: 10g

- Sugar: 15g

- Portion size: 1 smoothie

Pineapple Ginger Turmeric Smoothie

Ingredients:

- 1 cup chopped pineapple

- 1 tablespoon grated ginger

- 1 teaspoon ground turmeric

- 1 cup coconut water

- 1 tablespoon honey or agave syrup (optional)

Instructions:

1. Combine all ingredients in a blender.

2. Blend until smooth and creamy.

3. Serve immediately.

Nutrition Information:

- Calories: 130

- Protein: 1g

- Carbohydrates: 32g

- Fat: 0g

- Fiber: 3g

- Sugar: 25g

- Portion size: 1 smoothie

Peach Spinach Smoothie with Flaxseeds

Ingredients:

- 1 cup fresh spinach
- 1 ripe peach, pitted and sliced
- 1/2 cup plain Greek yogurt
- 1 tablespoon ground flaxseeds
- 1/2 cup almond milk

Instructions:

1. Place all ingredients in a blender.
2. Blend until smooth and creamy.
3. Pour into glasses and enjoy.

Nutrition Information:

- Calories: 180
- Protein: 10g
- Carbohydrates: 25g
- Fat: 6g
- Fiber: 5g
- Sugar: 15g
- Portion size: 1 smoothie

Kiwi Mango Smoothie with Chia Seeds

Ingredients:

- 2 ripe kiwis, peeled and diced
- 1 cup chopped mango
- 1 tablespoon chia seeds
- 1/2 cup coconut water
- Juice of 1 lime

Instructions:

1. Combine all ingredients in a blender.
2. Blend until smooth and creamy.
3. Serve immediately.

Nutrition Information:

- Calories: 160
- Protein: 3g
- Carbohydrates: 35g
- Fat: 3g
- Fiber: 8g
- Sugar: 20g
- Portion size: 1 smoothie

Orange Carrot Ginger Smoothie

Ingredients:

- 1 large carrot, peeled and chopped
- 1 orange, peeled and segmented
- 1 tablespoon grated ginger
- 1/2 cup orange juice
- 1/2 cup water

Instructions:

1. Place all ingredients in a blender.
2. Blend until smooth and creamy.
3. Pour into glasses and enjoy.

Nutrition Information:

- Calories: 120
- Protein: 2g
- Carbohydrates: 28g
- Fat: 1g
- Fiber: 6g
- Sugar: 18g
- Portion size: 1 smoothie

Beet Berry Smoothie with Hemp Seeds

Ingredients:

- 1 small beet, peeled and diced
- 1 cup mixed berries (such as strawberries, raspberries, blueberries)
- 1 tablespoon hemp seeds
- 1/2 cup almond milk
- 1 tablespoon honey or maple syrup (optional)

Instructions:

1. Combine all ingredients in a blender.
2. Blend until smooth and creamy.
3. Serve immediately.

Nutrition Information:

- Calories: 150
- Protein: 5g
- Carbohydrates: 25g
- Fat: 4g
- Fiber: 7g
- Sugar: 15g
- Portion size: 1 smoothie

Avocado Kale Smoothie with Matcha

Ingredients:

- 1/2 ripe avocado
- 1 cup chopped kale
- 1 teaspoon matcha powder
- 1 tablespoon honey or agave syrup
- 1 cup coconut water

Instructions:

1. Place all ingredients in a blender.
2. Blend until smooth and creamy.
3. Pour into glasses and enjoy.

Nutrition Information:

- Calories: 200
- Protein: 5g
- Carbohydrates: 25g
- Fat: 10g
- Fiber: 7g
- Sugar: 15g
- Portion size: 1 smoothie

Watermelon Mint Smoothie

Ingredients:

- 2 cups cubed seedless watermelon
- 1/4 cup fresh mint leaves
- 1/2 cup coconut water
- Juice of 1 lime
- 1 tablespoon honey or agave syrup (optional)

Instructions:

1. Place all ingredients in a blender.
2. Blend until smooth and creamy.
3. Pour into glasses and garnish with mint leaves if desired.
4. Serve immediately.

Nutrition Information:

- Calories: 90
- Protein: 1g
- Carbohydrates: 22g
- Fat: 0g
- Fiber: 1g
- Sugar: 18g
- Portion size: 1 smoothie

Mixed Berry Protein Smoothie with Almond Milk

Ingredients:

- 1 cup mixed berries (strawberries, raspberries, blueberries)
- 1 scoop vanilla protein powder
- 1 cup unsweetened almond milk
- 1 tablespoon almond butter
- 1 teaspoon honey or maple syrup (optional)

Instructions:

1. Combine all ingredients in a blender.
2. Blend until smooth and creamy.
3. Pour into glasses and serve immediately.

Nutrition Information:

- Calories: 250
- Protein: 20g
- Carbohydrates: 25g
- Fat: 9g
- Fiber: 5g
- Sugar: 15g
- Portion size: 1 smoothie

Papaya Coconut Smoothie with Lime

Ingredients:

- 1 cup diced ripe papaya
- 1/2 cup coconut milk
- 1/2 cup coconut water
- Juice of 1 lime
- 1 tablespoon honey or agave syrup (optional)

Instructions:

1. Place all ingredients in a blender.
2. Blend until smooth and creamy.
3. Pour into glasses and serve immediately.

Nutrition Information:

- Calories: 180
- Protein: 2g
- Carbohydrates: 30g
- Fat: 7g
- Fiber: 4g
- Sugar: 20g
- Portion size: 1 smoothie

CONCLUSION

As the final chapter unfolds, it's evident that this book is more than just a collection of recipes; it's a beacon of hope and possibility for those navigating the complex landscape of dietary management. Each recipe has been carefully crafted with both taste and blood sugar control in mind, ensuring that every meal contributes to a balanced and fulfilling lifestyle.

From the vibrant hues of breakfast smoothie bowls to the comforting aroma of dinner simmering on the stove, every dish serves as a reminder that managing Type 1 Diabetes doesn't mean sacrificing flavor or enjoyment. It's about embracing a new way of eating that nourishes both body and soul.

As we bid farewell to these pages, let us carry forth the knowledge gained within, armed with the tools and inspiration to create delicious, diabetes-friendly meals that ignite joy and vitality in our daily lives. May this cookbook serve as a steadfast companion on your journey to optimal health and well-being, reminding you that with a bit of creativity and determination, anything is possible.

In closing, remember that the power to thrive lies within each and every one of us. Let us embrace this newfound culinary adventure with open hearts and eager taste buds, knowing that with each meal we prepare, we're taking a step towards a brighter, healthier future.

www.ingramcontent.com/pod-product-compliance
Lightning Source LLC
Chambersburg PA
CBHW061640250726
48659CB00004B/1314